OTHER BOOKS BY THE AUTHOR

*Pediatrics: Some Uncommon Views on Some
Common Problems*

*Professionally Speaking: Public Speaking for Health
Professionals*

*Oratorio Para Profesionales de la Salud
(Professionally Speaking)*

*Medical Writing 101: A Primer for Health
Professionals*

Parenthood: Laugh and Understand Your Child

Ethical Problems in Pediatrics: A Dozen Dilemmas

*Effective Medical Communication
An Anthology of Columns from The DO Magazine*

Looking Back . . . at SECOM

Practicing for Practice

*Melnick on Writing
An Anthology of Columns from the American Medical Writers Association*

*Osteopathic Tales
Stories tracing one DO's travel along the path of the Osteopathic Profession
from Rejection and Discrimination to Recognition and Acceptance*

MONOGRAPHS

So you've been asked to speak . . .

Sandy, We Love You
(with Anita Melnick)

Who Will I Tell?

Giving Your Child Medication...*Safely*

A practical handbook for parents

Arnold Melnick, DO, MSc, DHL (Hon.), FACOP

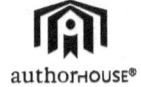

authorHOUSE®

AuthorHouse™ LLC
1663 Liberty Drive
Bloomington, IN 47403
www.authorhouse.com
Phone: 1-800-839-8640

Published by AuthorHouse   10/28/2013

ISBN: 978-1-4918-3024-6 (sc)
ISBN: 978-1-4918-3025-3 (e)

Library of Congress Control Number: 2013919267

Any people depicted in stock imagery provided by Thinkstock are
models, and such images are being used for illustrative purposes only.
Certain stock imagery © Thinkstock.

This book is printed on acid-free paper.

Table of Contents

Acknowledgement

I am indebted to

Scott Swigart, PharmD, Dean

Wegmans School of Pharmacy

St. John Fisher College

Rochester, NY

for his helpful support and careful review
of the first draft of this book

Dedication

To my late and wonderful wife

Anita

whose tremendous love and unending support

continues to inspire me even today

as it did throughout our lives together

Preface

I intend here to create a handbook for parents about the drugs they give their children, whether prescription or over-the-counter. My intention is for this book to answer their "little" questions (which could turn out to be big questions), to be able to have a reference, for example, on how to administer bad-tasting medicine, what mixes with what, and all the questions that go beyond the "take one pill three times a day" or "give one teaspoon every four hours" instructions.

So, the purposes of this book are:

1. To help parents understand their children's prescriptions
2. To help parents administer their children's prescriptions for maximum effectiveness, convenience and safety

3. To help parents in their use of over-the-counter (non-prescription) medication for children
4. To present applicable scientific information clearly and concisely.

There are really three reasons for creating such a book. First, there are very few helpful references like this for parents about their children and medicines. Second, dosages for children are sometimes inexact and difficult to calculate because medicines for adults are carefully researched in every aspect long before they are put on the market, whereas dosages for children are to a large extent inferred from the adult findings. And third, time pressures, changes in practice patterns and other factors have put doctors and pharmacists into a position where they cannot always put together sufficient time to give careful and precise instructions and fully answer parents' questions, or potential questions.

[An aside to all children: May you rarely need medication, but when you do, may you get the fullest benefit possible . . . safely]

Part One

WHAT PARENTS SHOULD KNOW

Chapter One

THIS BOOK AND YOU

This book was not made to read and put away; it is not like a novel. Looking at this book and reading sections that interest you would be the first step in your being able to have full control over the medications your children take. But after that, this book should become a reference and guidebook because it will answer so many questions that so many parents have—questions that sometimes are not answered by other sources or for questions that arise at a later date. The concern is that children, who do benefit greatly from pharmaceutical progress, should have an opportunity to get full effect from any medication they may take, without it endangering their health or life.

This book, written by an experienced pediatrician

with some input from an excellent doctor of pharmacy, will fill gaps in your knowledge of the administering of medication to your children. It should answer the questions that mothers and fathers would ask if they had the opportunity, and answer those questions they should ask, even if they are afraid to ask or forget to ask.

In all cases, the ultimate authorities on the medication your child is taking are your physician and your pharmacist. Questions not answered in this book should be referred to them and don't be afraid to ask! If you think there is any conflict between the advice given in this book and what you believe your physician or pharmacist has told you, do not hesitate to go back to either the physician or the pharmacist before giving medication to your child. They will appreciate it.

There are several things that this book is not meant to do

It is not meant to replace your physician or pharmacist. The ultimate authority for medication information for your child is one or both of those professionals. Never hesitate to call on them when there is a question.

It is not meant to be used in any way during the hospitalization of a child. Parents do not administer medication when a child is hospitalized. That is a special situation that requires a cooperative arrangement among the hospital, the physician, the parent, and the child. Some of things in this book might be applicable, but this book should never be used for that purpose. It is purely a book to be used in the home treatment of children. In hospitalization situations, consult your doctor.

It is not an emergency handbook. Emergencies, like hospitalization, are a special situation and should be dealt with directly between you and your physician. Drugs, medication and treatment in emergencies are not within the scope of this book. In emergencies involving ingestion of medication, call your local Poison Control Center at once. But parents should have that number at their fingertips early and always—it's an important emergency number. The telephone number is found in the front of your local telephone directory.

It is not meant for the purpose of training parents to treat or prescribe for their children. As I will say many times, whenever there is doubt or any question, consult your doctor or your pharmacist or both and follow their directions.

Chapter Two

TIPS AND RULES
FOR SAFETY

Health care professionals distinguish two kinds of medication (whether for children or adults): those ordered by the physician by prescription (called prescription medication) and those for which a prescription is not required, called over-the-counter medication (OTC).

In the latter category, often included are so-called "natural products" such as herbs and similar substances. Discussion on the natural products is beyond the scope of this book, but I would urge you to check with your physician or pharmacist before giving these products to your children. Although many reports give glowing recommendations to "natural products", most "natural products" are not regulated by the federal Food and Drug Administration, and they may not be standardized as to contents or dosage. For most of them, there are no accurate records or research reports about conflicts with other medications a child may be taking or possible unwanted and undesirable side effects. Precaution is the watchword—check first before giving such "medications" to children. "Natural" does not necessarily mean "safe".

On the other hand, OTC medications other than "natural products"—are standardized and approved by the federal Food and Drug Administration and thus allowed to be sold without prescription. However, FDA approval applies *only* if they are used according to the package instructions for indications, age of patient, dosage and dose intervals. Within these bounds, the medication is considered to be safe but its effectiveness is not guaranteed, nor can you be sure that it is the indicated medication for your child's illness. Parents are urged to conform to all label instructions on OTC products.

In the case of prescription medication, I have attempted in this book to provide parents with an understanding of prescriptions, with background on the best utilization of such prescriptions and with the best possible help in the home administration of those prescriptions. In the case of OTC products (such things as nose drops, ear drops, cough medicines, aspirin and other pain relievers, and other medicines) I have attempted to provide some background to complement the care of the physician or to make for better utilization of the prescription.

One of the most difficult decisions for a parent occurs when a child is ill but does not appear ill enough to consult a doctor. While it is never wrong to see your doctor when a child is sick, there are a number of instances in which parents often use OTC medication for minor complaints and illnesses in their children. Among these are mild pain (perhaps due to a bruise or a bump), colds, allergies, nasal stuffiness, mild cough, rashes and similar non-threatening illnesses. Most of the time, parents recognize when there is a serious illness or one that might become serious, and they call the physician. When, then, should you use OTC medication? Or, more importantly, when should you *not* use them? While it cannot be defined precisely, OTC medication should *never* be used in anything that is a severe or unusual complaint, or is potentially a serious illness, or could be a serious illness or you are not sure about. And I would personally add: *never* for a child younger than 2 or 3 years of age unless told to do so by a physician.

When considering OTC products, be sure to check with the pharmacist before making your purchase so that he or she can advise you whether it is appropriate medication for your child, whether it is to be used for the problem being treated, whether it conflicts with medication your child is taking or whether you should consult your physician first.

Precautions and Safety Hints

Several things should be kept in mind always for both prescription and for OTC medication. I offer here several general guides and some Do's and Don'ts to help ensure safe use of these products.

General Precautions

- Beware of self-diagnosis. If you are not absolutely sure about what is going on, consult your doctor or pharmacist.

- Always contact your child's physician *before* administering any medication.

- Always stick strictly to the directions on the bottle—unless instructed otherwise by your physician or pharmacist.

- Do not renew a prescription without your doctor's orders. Similarly, do not buy additional OTC medication beyond the first purchase without professional guidance. Parents sometimes do this with OTC laxatives or cold medicines. Persistence of symptoms always requires your physician's attention.

- Be very careful with OTC medication for coughs and colds. More than 100 of them contain DMX (dextramethorphan). This is a serious narcotic that is dangerous for children unless ordered by your physician. If there is a teenager in your house, it could be an attractive nuisance because that teenager may be tempted to experiment with drugs or may already be started and searching for more "supplies".

- A number of liquid OTC products contain alcohol (usually called elixirs) and obviously should never be given to children, unless ordered by a health professional. If your physician does order such medicine, keep a running record, in a separate location, of the amount remaining in the bottle after each dose. This serves as a double-check on the accuracy of your dosing. And it is especially valuable if there is a teenager in the house.

- Do not refrigerate a bottle of medicine unless the label says to do so. It may change the therapeutic effect.

- Never give a small child aspirin if there is a viral condition, for example, a cold. This may cause Reye's Syndrome, a potentially life-threatening illness. Depend solely, for a small child, on your physician's recommendation.

- Never put medicine in a bottle other than its original container. It may confuse you in identifying medication and inexact dosing may occur.

- Usually medication for small children will come in child-proof containers. If not, ask for them.

- Always keep medication out of the reach of small children. When going to a medicine cabinet, be absolutely sure you have the correct bottle—be sure there is enough light available to read the label and double-check the name and dates and dosage—<u>every time</u>.

- Observe expiration dates meticulously—never exceed them.

- For exact dosages, use calibrated measuring devices and not household utensils. They are not expensive and your pharmacist will often supply them. Ask for them when picking up the prescription.

- At any time, if a child begins wheezing or has difficulty breathing or problems swallowing or has any abnormal swelling after taking medication, whether prescription or OTC, call 911 at once. This probably represents an extreme allergic (and possible life-threatening) situation. Do not wait "to see how he or she will do."

Especially for prescriptions

- Discard all left-over medication. It should not be used because it may not maintain its strength, or the child's medical diagnosis may not be the same.

- On medication your doctor may have told you to keep, always check the expiration date before using.

- Never give a child someone else's medication— *even if you think the medical condition is the same.* Let your doctor decide that.

Especially for OTC medications

- Only use medication that is specifically made for children. Trying to adjust an adult dose for a child is fraught with danger.

- Do not deviate from any instructions on the label.

- Do not hesitate to ask your pharmacist anything about medication

And, finally, and probably most important:

Do not try to memorize or remember these important precautions. But, every time your child needs medication, consult this list again (and again)—to be safe, to be sure and not to be sorry.

Chapter Three

WHY ARE CHILDREN DIFFERENT?

Children are not small adults!

In almost all instances, if you simply reduce the adult dose of a particular medication proportionately to body weight differences between the adult and the child, the medication may not produce the same results. It may become an overdose or an under-dose. There is good reason for this possibility.

First, you must understand the differences between the body function of adults and children. Physiology is the study of the way a person's body actually operates. It refers to the function of organ systems in our body such as heart and blood, stomach and intestines, kidneys, liver, brain, and even the skin. Pharmacology is the study of the way the human body reacts to medication and how the medication behaves in the body. Each one of the organ systems has an effect on how a medication behaves in the body. They control how much of a medication gets into the body, that is, how much is absorbed (absorption), how it is distributed in the body (distribution) and how the body eliminates the medication (elimination or clearance). Based on these functions, we try to determine how much of a medication we should give and how often we give it.

Both physiology and pharmacology in a child are different from those in an adult! So we cannot simply treat children as small adults.

The rest of this chapter is dedicated to giving parents an understanding of how drugs work and is not intended to train you in their use.

How Drugs are Absorbed (Absorption)

There are only a few ways for a medication to get into the body. They are:

orally—when the medication is swallowed

intramuscularly (abbreviated as IM)—injected into a muscle

subcutaneously (abbreviated as SQ)—injected just under the skin

intravenously (abbreviated as IV)—injected directly into the blood stream

inhalation—when the medication is breathed in or inhaled

topically—when the medication is applied to the skin or directly introduced into bodily openings, for example, ears, eyes or nose.

Injected medications, whether intramuscular, subcutaneous or intravenous, are rarely used at home, *unless* the parent is specifically trained. In this book, we will deal mainly with the other modes of administration.

In general, medications that are administered to children by most of these routes are absorbed equally as well as in adults. The significant difference is in medications administered by injection into the muscle (intramuscular); these are almost always given by a trained professionals. A few words may help you understand this:—Young children have significantly less muscle mass than adults and the blood flow to those muscles can be much different because they do not use the muscles as much as adults. Until a child starts walking, the gluteal muscles (the main muscles of the buttocks) are undeveloped and the muscles of the upper arm and shoulder (the deltoid muscle) remain underdeveloped until after three years of age, even though used frequently in activities. Therefore, your health professional will usually avoid these sites until the child is at least three years of age. Even then the maximum volume (the total amount to be injected) of medication is very limited. If an intramuscular injection is needed in a child less than three years old, the mid-thigh is usually the site of choice.

How drugs are spread through the body (Distribution)

Once the medication is absorbed into the body, it is then distributed throughout the body. Usually, the medication is absorbed, directly or ultimately, into the blood and in turn is carried throughout the body, but sometimes unevenly. A medication does not "know where to go" and actually, it usually goes everywhere, as explained in Chapter Three. The chemical make-up of the medication will determine how much of the drug gets into the blood. The volume of blood an individual has, the percentage of that blood that is water (both of these are very similar among individuals), and the chemical properties of the medication all play a role in determining how much of a medication is given (the dose). Children, especially young children, tend to have a much higher proportion of water in their blood and body. This is one of the significant differences between children (especially young children) and adults; it is used when determining the correct dose of a medication. Also, this helps to explain why adult doses can not just be modified for weight differences in children and still get the same therapeutic results. Or why one child's (or adult's) medication should never be used for another child.

How drugs are eliminated from the body (Elimination)

As the medication circulates throughout the body, the body will begin to get rid of the medication; this is called elimination or clearance. Elimination of a medication from the body will occur in one of two ways: 1. the body may eliminate the medication unchanged into the urine (through the kidneys) after it has done its work; 2. the body may chemically change the medication in the liver (this process is called metabolism) to an inactive substance and then eliminate the inactive substance through the urine (some small amounts may be eliminated through other routes). The ability to eliminate medications in the urine is significantly reduced in the first year of life but after that is similar to adults during most of childhood. In treating infants with drugs that are known to be eliminated through the kidneys, medical professionals take special care.

The liver metabolism of medications varies significantly throughout childhood. Metabolism is slower compared to adults during the first two to three months of life and from then until puberty, it increases to average adult values. This difference in elimination at various ages of childhood has a significant influence on how much and how often a medication is given. For example, a medication that is eliminated by the liver might be given three times a day in an adult but may only be given one or two times a day in a newborn and maybe four times a day in a seven- or eight-year old. Again, this difference in the "physiology" of children makes it difficult to adjust an adult dose based only on weight and get the desired results. The adjustment of doses should only be done by a physician or pharmacist. If you attempt to guess or calculate a child's dose, the result may be an overdose or under-dose.

During childhood many of these organ systems are changing both in structure and function. Since they are changing, how a medication reacts will be different in newborns, infants, toddlers, school-age children, and adolescents. Theophylline, for example, is a medication sometimes used in infants for a breathing disorder called apnea (a temporary cessation of breathing) and in children and adults for asthma. It is a good example of how physiology affects how much and how often we give a medication. Infants treated for apnea require very small doses (even after adjusting for the difference in body weight) given only once or twice a day because children do not eliminate (metabolize) theophylline as well as older children or adults. After the age of 2 years, a child being treated for asthma will require much higher doses (again, compared on a weight basis) and given 4 times a day because children eliminate theophylline much faster than either infants or adults. Another good example of how age and physiology affect medications is chloramphenicol. Chloramphenicol

(Chloromycetin) is an antibiotic that was once used to treat, among other things, a very serious illness in children called meningitis (an infection of the brain and spinal cord) and sometimes other serious infections. Fortunately, oral Chloromycetin is no longer on the market. The correct dose for a five-year old would produce serious toxicities in a one-month old infant even when adjusted on a weight basis. The difference is in how the chloramphenicol is eliminated from the body at different ages.

Orphan Drugs

The federal Food and Drug Administration (FDA) has the responsibility of approving all medications— whether for adults or children before they go on the market. The FDA requires all medications to be tested to make sure that they do what they are intended to do (efficacy) and that they are safe, before they are approved to be used in the United States. These tests will determine (among other things) the correct dose and how often to give that dose. Before a manufacturer can advertise or give dosing information (even to physicians) for a medication used in children, it must first do extensive research in children. This research in children is often very difficult and expensive.

Because children use fewer medications and lesser amounts of those medications, it is not uncommon for a manufacturer not to do the needed studies in children because the overwhelming time required and the cost make it prohibitive. Therefore, many medications will not have a "labeled indication for children", which means no studies were done to determine the optimal dosing in children.

In fact, only about *25%* of all medications used in adults have a labeled indication for children. This does not mean that the medication may not be used for children, only that a scientific dosage has not been determined. In this situation the medication is referred to as a "therapeutic orphan" or an "orphan drug". This absence of research also occurs in drugs for very rare diseases (in either children or adults) where there are so few cases that it would be too expensive to do the studies to develop the medications and so few patients who would use them, so manufacturers cannot justify the cost (the FDA has recently started to provide cost incentives and grants to do this type of research). Any use of these drugs might be risky but must always be determined by your physician or your pharmacist.

Because so few medications have FDA-approved

dosing guidelines for children, there are some ways to estimate a dose for a child from established adult doses (simple weight differences are not enough). These methods generally employ calculating a dose based upon a ratio between a child's actual values and standard adult values for weight, age, or surface area **of** the body. Methods that use weight or age, are not generally reliable as they do not take into consideration the difference in the child's physiology or basic ability to use the medication. Methods that use body surface area provide a more reliable dose. When no labeled indication exists, physicians and pharmacists may use formulas which take into consideration height, weight, body surface, physiological differences, considerations of the illness being treated or any combination of these. What is important for parents to remember is that calculations for orphan drugs must never be done by parents, only by physicians or pharmacists. Children of the same age are not all the same weight, and children of the same weight are not all the same age.

Breast Milk-Transmitted Medication

A number of medications prescribed for nursing mothers may pass through her body and be excreted in the breast milk. As well, a number of medications are not excreted in the milk. Those excreted in the milk will enter the infant's body and can affect the infant. Even in the normal infant, this may cause difficulties. Every nursing mother should check with her obstetrician or pediatrician to determine the status of medication that she may be taking and to ask for advice about it in view of her nursing an infant.

Especially when the infant is taking medication, the nursing mother should check with her physician to be absolutely certain that nothing she is ingesting for herself (prescription or over-the-counter) comes through in the breast milk, possibly augmenting, interfering with or counteracting any medication being given directly to the baby—even affecting the baby directly. This is very important and every mother should be alert to remind her physician that she is breast feeding whenever she is put on medication or whenever her infant is put on medication.

Special Situations

A word needs to said about two special situations: Fetal Alcohol Syndrome and effects of cigarette smoking. Neither is specifically tied in with breast milk-transmitted drugs, but they might be connected, and they are serious conditions relating to a pregnant woman and her fetus.

Fetal Alcohol Syndrome. In this condition, if the pregnant mother ingests "abnormal' amounts of alcohol during her pregnancy, a number of malformations may occur in the fetus. such as growth retardation, small-sized head, abnormal eye structures and cardiac and orthopedic defects. In almost every instance, the child has mental retardation, perhaps the most serious of the findings. Unfortunately, with present-day knowledge, we cannot establish whether there is a safe alcohol intake for a pregnant woman, nor at what stage of the pregnancy the alcohol has its most serious effect. Thus, the strong advice, very strong, is that a pregnant woman should not drink alcohol of any kind—beer, wine or hard liquor—during her pregnancy. The emphasis is on *none,* not even a little bit, and regardless of what form the alcohol is in. The danger to the fetus is too great.

We do know that in nursing mothers, alcohol will come through the breast milk if the infant nurses within three hours of the alcohol ingestion. It has been found that breast-fed infants, in this circumstance, consume 25% less milk during that three-hour period. Once again, the strongest advice is for nursing mothers to avoid alcohol.

Cigarette smoking. While we know many of the effects on the fetus of mother's smoking, we cannot pin down the exact mechanisms and their timing,—whether the causation is the nicotine, the mother's inhalation of smoke, blood transmission of harmful substances or dangerous effects. We do know that babies of pregnant mothers who smoke tend to be lighter in birth weight and that the incidence of stillbirths, spontaneous abortion and death shortly after birth is higher in smokers than in non-smokers. Once again, for maximum good health, the advice must be:

Do not smoke when pregnant! And just for good measure, try to avoid second-hand smoke during the pregnancy, because we know the harmful effects of this at all ages.

Chapter Four

HOW DRUGS WORK
IN CHILDREN

Doctors and pharmacists have a complicated scientific system—called Pharmacology, which we will not discuss here—for figuring out exactly how a drug works in the body, what organs it affects and how it achieves its purpose. However, from a purely practical standpoint—a parent's viewpoint—to help in understanding the medications you give your children, you must consider two things:

No drug or medication has a single effect

You must understand that all authorities agree that no medication has only a single effect on the patient's body; parents must always keep that in mind.

It is one of the most important facts in the prescribing, administering and evaluating of all medicines. For example, if your physician gives your child an injection for an acute attack of asthma, the drug does not just flow to a specific spot and stop the attack of asthma. It also has an effect on the circulatory system, it has an effect on skin temperature, on the blood flow to the skin. In other words, the medication goes to *all* parts of the body, and may affect any or all of them.

Suppose you give your 12-year old child who has a headache an aspirin tablet. The aspirin dissolves and spreads throughout his body. When it reaches his head or wherever the headache originates, it will relieve that symptom. In fact, that headache might be coming from something local, that is, directly from the head where the ache is felt (as in a bump), or from some distant problem or from changes in the body metabolism (such as an infection or fever). The aspirin relieves the headache because it diffuses through and affects all the structures of the body regardless of where they are. It probably will even relieve a pain from a different source in another separate location.

Another result of taking the aspirin—or any other drug—is its production of other symptoms. This is called a side-effect. One of the negative side effects of aspirin is that it can cause direct local irritation of the stomach lining. This could create nausea or other problems.

Thus, medications frequently have side-effects; that is something not always recognized by parents. When those side-effects are extreme, it is called toxicity because it presents potential danger. Ignoring side-effects can put the child at risk. Always report these to your doctor.

Some medications are manufactured with multiple ingredients for different aspects of the treatment of a specific condition, say a cold or cough. Each ingredient is there for a reason: one is usually for the main therapeutic effect, one or more to bolster the main ingredient, one or more to counter some side-effect of the main ingredient, or some other purposeful reasons. Obviously, if the medicine has four or five ingredients, each of those will have its own effects and side-effects. The total impact on the body—and the dangers—will therefore be multiple because there will be effects from each of the ingredients.

Physicians constantly face the problem of the

side-effects or the possible "bad" effects on a child of administering any medication. That leads to mothers' occasional complaints that "The medication did what the doctor told me it would do, but Tommy now has several new symptoms since he has been taking the medicine. I can't decide whether they are new symptoms or a new illness." Actually, it may simply be the side-effect of the medication. Generally, stopping the medicine will shortly end the side-effect, but it is always best to check with your physician or pharmacist to find out.

The medication does not know where it is going

To believe that a particular medicine, whether it is a prescription or an over-the-counter remedy, heads directly for the affected area, and the affected area alone, is incorrect. Imagine a glass of water. Into it you put five or six drops of food coloring. Immediately, or within a few minutes, the entire glass of water has become tinted with the color that was added. In other words, the coloring has dispersed throughout the entire glass of water. The same phenomenon occurs with medication entering the body.

Let's take an example. Susie breaks out in an

allergic skin rash over her arm. Your doctor diagnoses it as a contact dermatitis, that is, an allergic reaction to something with which her skin has come in contact. In some cases your physician may prescribe an antihistamine by mouth, a reasonable treatment, and that medication will take the rash away. However, since we already understand that the antihistamine will be generally dispersed throughout the entire body, it will have the same effect as it would have when you use that same antihistamine for a respiratory allergy. For one example, Susie will have some drying of her nasal tissues, even though she has no problem or complaint about the nose. If you use that medication for a long period of time or in large doses, that dryness will become annoying to her, and the child can be said to have a side-effect of the medication.

Sometimes a side-effect is strong enough or important enough that the physician will order the medicine discontinued, especially if the side-effect symptoms outweigh the benefit of the medication. Sometimes a medication is so important that the child—and you—just have to put up with the inconvenience, as long as it does not endanger the child. This is a decision the doctor should make, but you must notify the physician or pharmacist of any unusual effects or reactions which occur in your child. Because of these considerations, your doctor must give very careful consideration for every prescription for any drugs or pharmaceuticals. It is not simply a matter of picking the right drug for the particular symptoms or disease. It also means picking one with the least side-effects while not minimizing the therapeutic results. Without understanding this background, it might be difficult for parents to understand how doctors make their choice.

In determining the dose of the medication for your child, your physician will have taken note of your child's body size, weight and activity levels. All of these influence the amount of medication to be given and the rate at which it may be metabolized or used up.

KINDS OF DRUGS

Medical science does not have a cure for every disease, or even a cure for every symptom, so not all medication cures, whether a prescription or an over-the-counter drug. Your doctor may administer drugs to achieve one or several effects, and it will help you to understand the medications your child takes if you have some idea of how we classify drugs by their general effectiveness:

Those that cure

These are the drugs which actually cure a particular disease or symptom. Among the finest examples are antibiotics. A clear example is the use of penicillin for the treatment of streptococcal sore throat ("strep throat") or the previously discussed and no longer used chloramphenicol (Chloromycetin) in meningitis (Chapter 2). The penicillin has a direct effect on the bacteria that are growing in the child's throat (and has a similar effect on other tissues whether or not there is streptococci in those other tissues). The proper amount of the penicillin given for the proper amount of time will generally kill off the bacteria and thus eradicate the "strep throat". This is curing a condition, but the number of medicines available which actually cure diseases or illnesses is limited.

Those that relieve symptoms

Your physician may use certain medications when there is no drug that cures the disease but orders them given to assist in the alleviation of symptoms. Sometimes they are used in addition to the curative drug while the cure-agent gets the time it needs to do the work. Another simple example is the use of aspirin in the average simple headache of unknown cause. This is a situation in which there is no apparent reason for the headache and therefore no curative medication. Taking aspirin will relieve the symptom and if there is no other disease or illness, the body will correct itself and the problem will end. For a second illustration, let's go back to the "strep throat". The penicillin will cure the illness, but your doctor may also advise aspirin to relieve the discomfort of the child (the sore throat) and the fever until the penicillin completes its work. This is symptomatic use.

Those that support the body in healing

This is treatment that does not directly affect the disease or relieve symptoms. It is important to understand that most medications have an effect that helps the body, but in the long run it is necessary for the body to "cure itself," that is, to exert its immunological or recuperative powers for curing. If those powers are diminished or lacking, the medication will not be successful. Certain medications are valuable for providing support to ill patients and for aiding their bodies to fight off the illness. Examples are fluids, nutrition, vitamins and similar aids. After all, it's the child's body ultimately which fights off and defeats the disease, and we want to give it all the help we can.

Another way to think of the effect of drugs on children is in terms of when and how they exert their effect.

You can consider those drugs that have an instantaneous or immediate effect. This is essentially a curative function. For example, the use of epinephrine (Adrenalin) in the treatment of asthma. It is given by injection for speed of action, and does its job in a matter of minutes, sometimes seconds. It stops the attack of asthma and in effect cures the attack. However, it only cures that particular attack and has no real effect in the long term or in curing the underlying illness or in preventing other attacks.

You can consider those drugs that have a short-term effect. These, too, are curative. One of the best examples is the use of antibiotics as already discussed. They are given for a few days, and usually help the body to get rid of the infection. If re-infection occurs, additional antibiotic may have to be given, but they have no preventive effect.

You can consider those drugs that have a long-term effect. An example is replacement therapy. In a child with thyroid deficiency, the doctor will prescribe thyroid substance by mouth—over a very long period of time if the thyroid gland does not start to work again, even in some cases for a lifetime. It does not cure, but is replacement of a vital and necessary body substance that is lacking. Insulin is a similar product. Steroids are at times in the same category, supporting the body over a short- or long-term until the disease comes under control.

SIDE-EFFECTS AND DANGEROUS EFFECTS

As we have indicated, no drug has only a single effect. Therefore, even using a drug that does what it is supposed to, there are likely to be many other effects. Some of these, as we noted, are simply called side-effects, as they are not usually dangerous or harmful. They are merely moderate annoyances the patient has to endure in order to get the treatment effect. All drugs—prescribed or over-the-counter—have the potential of side-effects. Fortunately, these effects generally do not appear in all persons at all times. There are several types of side-effects:

1. Some of these side-effects appear immediately or almost immediately. As we pointed out, oral antihistamine used for a skin rash may give, for example, a very obvious dryness of the nose. If the dryness is not too uncomfortable, it may be necessary for the child to tolerate it in order to get the needed effect of the antihistamine on the rash.

2. Some side-effects are less apparent. Acetominophen (Tylenol), an example of one of our most popular over-the-counter drugs, is used for reduction of fever or alleviation of pain, and usually does its job well without any obvious difficulties. However, lurking in the background is the possibility that in cases of prolonged use of Tylenol or over-dosage of Tylenol, there are reports of liver problems. The patient will not be aware of this, as no signs or symptoms appear at the time the drug is being taken. Obviously, parents and physicians must always be aware of such possibilities.

3. A third side-effect might be called insidious or slow developing. In the days when

tetracycline (Terramycin) was a widely-used antibiotic, a number of young children were treated with Terramycin for their illnesses, with very successful results. It was not discovered until after the eruption of the second set of teeth (permanent teeth) in a large number of children that it was realized that Terramycin, given under the age of 6, had a tendency to stain the developing set of permanent teeth. This caused some children to have permanently yellowed teeth. Like Chloromycetin, it took many years to discover these latent side-effects. Fortunately, oral Chloromycetin is no longer available and the use of Terramycin is banned for children under 6 years of age.

4. A fourth dangerous side-effect is one which actually occurs in only a very small number of children, and therefore is difficult to diagnose. A most effective antibiotic is chloramphenicol (Chloromycetin), previously mentioned in Chapter 2. It can also have a horrendous side-effect: the destruction of red blood cells. However, this bad effect occurred only about once in 30,000 patients taking Chloromycetin,

meaning that a large number of doctors might treat a large number of patients over a period of time before the first case would be evident. Yet it is a serious enough side-effect that extreme care has to be taken in the use of the drug, as valuable as it is.

As each of these serious side-effects or toxic consequences was discovered, physicians became alerted to them and exerted extra care and attention with those drugs in order to reduce or eliminate the possibility of problems.

Physicians are continually alert to various side-effects, both simple and dangerous. In prescribing medication, they look not only for the best therapeutic drug but one which will have the minimum of side-effects, particularly the dangerous ones. If your child has an allergy or reaction to a medication, ask your doctor or pharmacist to put it in his or her record. You should be sure to inform any subsequent physician about it.

There is another instance in which special care needs to be exercised. Many times your physician might need to prescribe two drugs to your child simultaneously for two different conditions. It can happen that they may be incompatible, that is, the effect of one counteracts the effect of the other, in which case the planned-for therapeutic result does not occur. On the other hand, the effects of one might enhance the effect of the other, creating an additive effect, resulting in an overdose. Most physicians are alert to these possibilities and prescribe accordingly. Most frequently, this situation will arise in one of two situations: first, when the doctor is not made aware of other medications that have been prescribed for the child (for example, from another specialist), or the child is given an over-the-counter product which the doctor does not know about.

An instance of the enhancement danger is when a patient is on a blood thinner like warfarin (Coumadin) and absolutely must not take aspirin, not even one aspirin for a single headache, because the aspirin will add to the effects of the Coumadin and can lead to very serious bleeding problems. In cases like this, physicians and pharmacists will give verbal and written warnings to the patient such as, "Do not take this medicine with—" ".You must observe such warnings diligently.

It is not necessary for you as a parent to know or remember these various classifications. Nor is it necessary to know all the side-effects and toxicities of a number of drugs. As a parent, you should want to be aware of the side-effects of the specific drugs your child is taking (ask your doctor or pharmacist), especially if the drug is being taken for a long time. Report anything different or unusual immediately. This is being an informed parent.

Chapter Five

READING PRESCRIPTIONS & PRESCRIPTION LABELS

A prescription is a message from the physician to the pharmacist, giving instructions on which medication to dispense to your child, and what instructions to put on the prescription label about how to take the medicine. The prescription label is the information that is placed on the medication bottle providing information for the patient and parent about the medication and how to take the medicine.

Why would a section on prescriptions be included in a book like this, written for parents? Over the past years, the philosophy has grown that parents should take an active role in their child's medical care, sharing this responsibility with their doctors and pharmacists.

More and more people have started to take this active role because it helps them considerably and also helps their doctors. There are so many decisions that have to be made along the course of writing, filling and using a prescription that errors can occur in so many places. The more informed parents become, the more likely they will discover any errors along the way—and the child is that much safer.

Similarly, more and more parents are taking a greater role in the responsibility for their children's health. No one has suggested that parents learn how to write prescriptions, but it would be a very constructive aid if you know a few things about prescriptions to help you follow your child's medication progress, and prevent the occasional error.

Both prescription blanks and prescription labels, in real life, have a variety of forms and shapes. However, there is certain basic information that must appear, and does appear, on every one. For illustrative purposes, however, the examples and figures given here have been created to contain all that required information and to provide clarity to the readers.

A prescription (see Figure 1) consists of several parts (don't try to learn these names):

1. The top of the blank, containing name of the patient, address, age or date of birth, date written and sometimes gender or weight is added, if important

2. The superscription, containing the Recipe (indicated by the symbol Rx, which means "take")

3. The inscription, telling the pharmacist what medication to dispense, and how much

4. The subscription, which tells the pharmacist how to compound the medication or how to dispense it

5. The signature (usually abbreviated as Sig.), which gives directions for the patient (and is transferred to the prescription by the pharmacist), followed by the prescriber's signed name

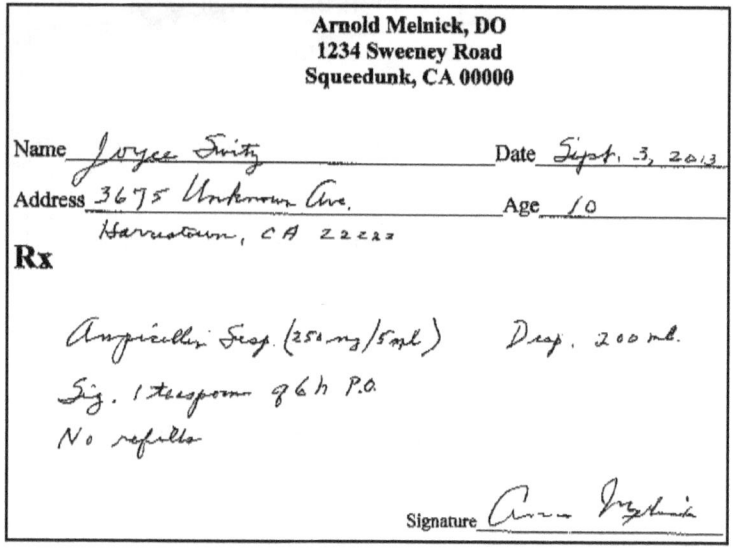

Arnold Melnick, DO
1234 Sweeney Road
Squeedunk, CA 00000

Name _Joyce Smity_   Date _Sept. 3, 2013_

Address _3675 Unknown Ave._   Age _10_
Harristown, CA 22222

Rx

Ampicillin Susp. (250 mg/5ml)   _Disp. 200 ml._
Sig. 1 teaspoon q 6 h P.O.
No refills

Signature _Arnold Melnick_

Figure 1

Look again at Figure 1. Following the Rx is the line
Ampicillin Susp. (250 mg/5 ml) PO

This tells the pharmacist to prepare a bottle of
Ampicillin Suspension which contains 250 milligrams
of the medication in each teaspoonful—given by mouth.
And it tells the pharmacist to give the patient 200 ml of
the mixture (40 doses).

Then, the prescription says on the next line:
Sig. 1 teaspoon q 6 hrs PO

This tells the pharmacist to label the prescription "one teaspoonful by mouth every 6 hours".

Some of the more commonly-used abbreviations you might see on a prescription are:

> Tsp—teaspoon
> Qd—once a day
> BID—twice a day
> TID—three times a day
> QID—four times a day
> qAM—every morning
> qHS—every night at bedtime

However, current thinking dictates that fewer and fewer abbreviations be used and the information should be written out. So great is the possibility for errors to occur that many hospitals today prohibit the use of such abbreviations. If you have any trouble understanding a prescription because of abbreviations, CONSULT YOUR PHRAMACIST OR PHYSICIAN IMMEDIATELY.

In the signature (Sig.), the physician may also add other directions, such as "after meals", "before meals", "with water" or other specific instructions.

Sometimes, the physician will use a brand name of a drug, instead of the medication name. You probably will not be able to identify it. Ask if you are not sure. Sometimes the manufacturer's name is added.

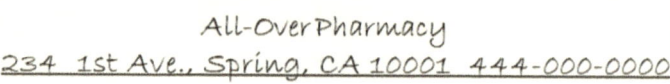

JOYCE SWITZ   3675 Blank Ave. Harristown, CA 22222

AMPICILLIN SUSPENSION (250 mg/5 ml)   Qty. 200 ml.
    Take one teaspoon by mouth every 6 hours

Dr. A. Melnick   Rx #123456   Sept. 3, 2013

No refills

Figure 2

A prescription label for the patient (see Fig. 2) consists of several parts but not necessarily in this order, varying with the pharmacy:

1. The name, address and phone number of the pharmacy

2. The patient's name and address

3. The name of the medication, the strength, and maybe the manufacturer

4. The directions for taking the medication, including the dose, route of administration and frequency

5. The prescription number, the physician's name, and the date

6. Quantity and refill information (how many times the pharmacist may refill the prescription without requiring another written prescription)

7. Auxiliary stickers

Figure 2 represents the label that would accompany the prescription in Figure 1. The information does not have to be in the same order—and often is not. The prescription number is how the pharmacy keeps a record of and files the original prescription. For a medication that has refills, the pharmacist can locate the original prescription and refill the medication according to this number. The directions are very important and tell the patient how to take the medication plus any special instructions such as "take at bedtime". The auxiliary stickers provide additional information about taking or storing the medication or other important instructions. Some of the commonest auxiliary stickers are:

Take with food or milk

Take with a full glass of water

Do not take with food

Swallow whole, do not chew or crush

May cause drowsiness, alcohol may intensify this effect.

Use care when operating a car or dangerous machinery.

Shake well before use

Keep refrigerated

Discard after   /   /

The value of knowing even limited amounts of information like this is multiple. Perhaps you thought the doctor said twice a day and the prescription seems to say three times a day. Check it with the doctor. Maybe you have a hard time deciphering whether it says "with food" or "without food". That may mean the pharmacist may also have a difficult time. Check it with the doctor and the pharmacist. The more you know, the more help you can be. The earlier that mistakes or confusion can be picked up, the safer it is for everyone.

It is most important that any unanswered questions, differences of opinion or misunderstandings be resolved before the prescription is dispensed and especially before the child is given any of the medication—not even the first dose. When in doubt, call your doctor or pharmacist.

Part Two

USE OF MEDICATIONS

Chapter Six

COMMON TREATMENTS FOR COMMON PROBLEMS

Common problems are those which occur with great frequency in children. Some require medication, some can be treated with non-prescription medication or even non-drug methods, some require both and some require neither. We will approach these common entities with a description of both methods. None of this is intended to replace or second-guess the ultimate decision-maker, your physician, and his/her colleague, your pharmacist. Serious illness or persistent symptoms or questionable situations should always be referred to one or both of them.

Trauma

This includes bumps, bruises, strains and sprains. More serious traumatic situations, for example, fractures, cuts, etc., absolutely require professional attention.

Because doctors and parents are accustomed to hearing children cry for a lot of little things, all of us tend to overlook the importance of the relief of pain as an important factor in trauma in children. The child who has been injured has pain just as much as the adult who has been injured. It is our duty, since children cannot express themselves in accurate terms about the amount of pain, to evaluate children's pain in relation to their injury. Fractures hurt, lacerations hurt, multiple abrasions hurt and contusions hurt. Therefore, your children should receive something almost immediately for the relief of their pain in addition to any local treatment. This not only makes them more comfortable (and usually more cooperative) but makes them understand that you care for them.

Very important in the treatment of the injured child is tender loving care and psychological support. How often these attentions are overlooked! Any adult who has ever been injured understands the amount of fright, fear, and anxiety caused by injury and often by any treatment which follows. If we, as adults, can realize those feelings that are in the mind of a child, who is less mature and less understanding, we might appreciate the intensity of the child's feelings. Your support when your child is injured is an absolutely necessary part of the treatment, and has an incalculably positive effect. Children should be handled gently and tenderly. Remember that they are "midgets" in a sea of "giants". Children must never be chastised for carrying on or for crying (or even for over-reacting, as sometimes happens) when they are injured. You or other adults never have justification for losing your temper with a traumatized child. Regardless of the child's behavior, you must always keep in mind that the child is terribly scared. If inappropriate behavior does occur, it can be discussed with the child sometime after the acute episode is over.

Adolescents are often overlooked in their need for the same support as small children. They have great problems with their body image. They are concerned about how they look, how they will grow, how they compare in body structure to other adolescents. And they are particularly concerned when a body part is injured.

Therefore, especially with adolescents, reassurance is necessary constantly, and it is most needed when the adult in charge is certain that the trauma will have no long-term effect on bodily appearance or function. Thus, adolescents need the same support and reassurance from adults as do smaller children. Many times, so do adults.

Although it is generally helpful in relieving pain, anti-pain medication does little toward curing or improving the actual healing process; however, it should always be used when the discomfort is more than mild. Thus, when a child falls and bumps his knee, aspirin or other pain-relief medication will not heal the knee any faster, but it will give some relief of pain. Aspirin should not be used in younger children and never if there is any kind of viral infection present; medication of choice would be acetaminophen (Tylenol), given according to age.

Non-pharmaceutical treatment might consist of the direct application of cold compresses (perhaps 20 minutes every hour) for the first 48 hours. This not only takes some of the pain away but reduces the swelling or keeps it from becoming excessive. At the end of 48 hours, you may switch to warm compresses (not hot) given in the same way. Some physicians prefer continuing the cold especially while there is swelling present. If there is a lot of swelling and it is in an extremity (i.e., a foot or a hand), elevate the affected extremity to help with drainage of the traumatized area. In an extremity injury, soaks are an alternative to compresses. Do not forget to rest the traumatized part; early on, use of an injured limb should be limited in order to help healing. And call your doctor for anything that looks unusual or that doesn't respond to treatment quickly enough.

Nasal Stuffiness or Mild Cold

Every cold does not need medication—and antibiotics will not cure or improve colds (they may cause additional troubles).

You might treat simple nasal stuffiness with the use of nose drops (or oral antihistamines or drying agents). These do not cure the cold, but do offer temporary relief of symptoms until the body rids itself of the illness or the viral infection has run its course.

For example, one effective non-pharmaceutical treatment for nasal stuffiness is an uncomplicated home remedy. Mix one-quarter teaspoon of ordinary table salt (measured accurately) and one-quarter teaspoon of baking soda (bicarbonate of soda, *not* baking *powder)* into 8 ounces of warm water. This mixture can be used as often as needed—several drops in each nostril. Be sure to clear the nose as much as possible before instilling the drops, as described in Nose Drops (Chapter 5).

When using these solutions, they should be made up freshly every day. If you are using a dropper bottle with its own dropper, replacing the dropper in the bottle after each use will generally maintain sterility. But you must be careful not to touch the dropper to any other surface or to the nose of the child because it might pick up or spread infection. This means that if you are improvising with a dropper that does not fit directly into the bottle, be sure to wash the dropper carefully before each use.

The simplest pharmaceutical treatment for nasal stuffiness is probably the use of simple over-the-counter nose drops such as Neosynephrine 1/4% (or 1/8% in infants), using one drop (in infants) to three drops (in older children) in each nostril every four hours. For any other kind of nose drops, your physician or your pharmacist should be consulted.

All children with colds and with nasal stuffiness should be provided with plenty of fluids by mouth (water, fruit juices, sweet tea and clear liquids). Increasing fluid intake helps to dilute the nasal mucus and in many instances the child will not need much more. Increased intake of fluids is also recommended even in children who are getting nose drops or a doctor-prescribed medication.

Cough Medicines

These are among the most frequently sold over-the-counter medications. A large variety of such products is available, with varying ingredients and varying effects. The therapeutic value will vary from product to product and, in part, on the child's condition. The side-effects will vary likewise with what is in the medication. We strongly suggest that you consult with your physician or your pharmacist before purchasing cough medicines over-the-counter. There are some indications for some types of cough medicine, other indications for other types and in many instances there is no indication for any medicine. Choosing properly is a difficult task and you really need professional advice to decide.

Since most coughing is caused by the irritation of thick mucous secretions in the back of the throat, everything that has been said for the use of oral fluids in nasal congestion can be said doubly for children with cough. Room temperature liquids by mouth again are recommended—water, fruit juices, or weak tea. Patients need, above all, the extra fluids topically and internally. One of the most helpful aids is the use of vaporized water (no added medication is needed), which provides topical moisture. Old-fashioned steam may be used to moisten the air, but cold-air vaporizers and ultra-sonic vaporizers are available to provide better moisture and are safer. If the cough appears to be the result of post-nasal drip coming from a nasal passage stuffed with sticky secretions, frequent instillation of salt or salt-baking soda drops, followed by nasal aspiration with a bulb syringe will aid the child. Involvement of the sinuses causing heavy nasal drip, or a suspicion of sinusitis, calls for a visit to the physician.

Sore throat

Sore throat is most frequently a secondary effect from a cold or post-nasal drip. Medication (including antibiotics), whether prescription or over-the-counter, rarely cures, unless it is a specific bacterial infection, but may help ease the discomfort. In severe or persistent cases, your physician should decide whether there is a bacterial infection, as antibiotics may be effective, but only effective in bacterial infection. Since antibiotics have no effect on viral infections they should not be used. In fact, use of antibiotics may sensitize the child and create an allergy to that antibiotic. In mild sore throats, the younger child (under 4 years) will get some additional relief of symptoms from repeated sucking on lollipops. Hard sweet candy is also helpful, but because of age, the danger for younger children from choking is great. First, the sweetness coats the tissues and gives a soothing effect. Second, the frequent swallowing that follows helps eliminate discomfort and moves secretions along.

Children over 8 years of age will also respond to this but in addition may get some relief by gargling several times a day with warm salt water. The use of gargles or hard sweet candy may add an additional soothing effect in infected throats even when antibiotics are being given, as they may help relieve symptoms.

Earache

Earache or otitis media (the medical term for it) is one of the more common illnesses in childhood. It is characterized by the onset of irritability, fever, and pulling or tugging on the ear. It is not uncommon to have cold symptoms (nasal stuffiness or coughing and congestion) occur before the symptoms of the earache. It is estimated that 9 out of 10 children will have an earache by the time they are 7 years old and about 6 out of 10 children will have an earache by the time they are one year old. It is most common in children from 9 to 12 months of age. Young children (less than 7 years old) are more likely to get earache because the inner ear is still developing and changing. The tube (called the Eustachian tube) that connects the middle ear to the nasal cavity provides drainage of fluid from the middle ear. In young children, this tube is shorter and at a different angle than in adults which makes it more difficult to drain. Because of this poor drainage, it forms a place for infections to occur. As children grow older, the angle of this tube changes and provides for better drainage. As a result, the incidence of earaches in most children decreases dramatically after the age of 6 years.

The earache is usually an infection from bacteria. Because of this, it must be treated with antibiotics. In addition, it is not uncommon to use a nasal decongestant with or without ear drops to help relieve pain. It is very important that children with the symptoms of an earache see their physicians. To treat, a specific diagnosis must be made. The doctor must decide what antibiotics should be used, if any, and whether or not the ear needs surgical drainage. A major problem with infection of the middle ear is the danger that it can lead to permanent hearing loss. This could be a very serious problem because hearing loss in a young child can affect speech, language development, learning and behavior.

Vomiting and diarrhea

Vomiting and diarrhea are very common occurrences in childhood. They are among the most frequent complaints found in young children. While most cases of vomiting and diarrhea are simple and can be treated simply, we must never be fooled into forgetting that they can be potentially dangerous. You are never wrong in consulting your physician when this occurs.

However, many mothers are capable of handling the simple cases of vomiting or diarrhea, as long as they keep in mind that any worsening of symptoms, prolongation of symptoms, or appearance of new symptoms should lead to an immediate call to the child's physician.

These symptoms can also be secondary to such illnesses as viral respiratory infection, or simple bellyache (eating of wrong foods). If the vomiting or diarrhea is secondary to a true bacterial infection elsewhere, often in the throat, the major part of the child's care is the treatment of that infection, along with whatever additional supportive treatment you can give the gastrointestinal system. For this, you need the advice of your doctor.

Most often, vomiting or diarrhea is caused by direct irritation of the intestinal tract, whether stomach or intestines. Whether the cause is from a primary or secondary source, probably one of the most effective aids in any simple involvement of the intestinal tract is complete rest of the part involved. That is true of *any* part of the body, whether a bumped elbow or a sprained ankle or certainly of the intestinal tract. Generally, the best approach is to allow the body part to rest and recover spontaneously, being healed by nature.

As the bowel, upper or lower or both, is given a chance to quiet down and recuperate, the symptoms of a simple involvement will disappear in most instances in short order. It's easy to understand when you tell someone, "Rest your arm" or "Rest your ankle" after trauma, but how do you rest your intestinal tract? Simply by giving it the least amount of work to do: no foods, no milk products, no junk food, just the lightest intake (or none for a while) such as weak, sweet tea, followed by other clear liquids when tolerated.

In addition to the resting of the part, there are other considerations. For example, if the bowel is put at complete rest, that is, absolutely no food or drink, the patient may be in danger of becoming dehydrated or of being denied necessary nutrition. These two possible complications must therefore be considered along with the value of resting of the body part.

If you are treating a simple gastroenteritis, the first recommendation is that the child be given nothing whatsoever by mouth for anywhere from 4 to 8 hours, allowing the bowel to quiet down, followed by therapy to be described. If the case is very mild, this "starvation period" can be eliminated.

While the treatment described here is for uncomplicated vomiting or diarrhea, it may sometimes be used along with the therapy your doctor prescribes. However, your doctor's regimen is the one that should be used.

Vomiting

If a child is vomiting and has no diarrhea, no other symptoms and no fever (or at most, a very low grade fever), I usually recommend the use of small sips of weak, sweet tea. This provides a bland but helpful fluid in small enough quantities that it will not to be rejected by the stomach, because when the stomach is irritated, it will not tolerate large volumes, regardless of the fluid being used. Generally, our recommendation is one teaspoonful every 15 or 20 minutes to start. Even though this appears to be a small quantity, its steady repetition goes a long way in preventing or minimizing dehydration, especially if it is increased gradually, as directed.

Using this therapy does two other things. The use of sweetened tea gives the child small amounts of sugar over the course of day. Tea contains the chemical tannic acid, one of the most effective soothers of the mucous membrane lining of the intestine. Therefore the child is getting some nourishment from the sugar, an anti-inflammatory effect on the mucous membrane of the bowel, and a start on sufficient fluids to avoid dehydration. The procedure, which starts with that one teaspoonful every 15 or 20 minutes with a *slow* and gradual increase in the amounts taken. For example, we would prescribe, after four to six doses of the initial amount without recurrence of vomiting, an increase in the amount to two teaspoons every 15 or 20 minutes. After four to six of these doses are held down, you may increase the intake to three teaspoons or ½ ounce of tea every 15 to 20 minutes. Then the interval can be lengthened, and the dose increased, for example, 3/4 ounce of tea every 30 minutes for four or five successful doses, then gradually increase the amount and lengthen the interval. This is kept up for 24 to 48 hours. and almost invariably, the vomiting will have stopped shortly after the beginning of treatment. Meanwhile, you have given sufficient fluids and some calories but without irritating the gastrointestinal tract. Amounts given at any one dose should be based on the age and size of the child.

The success of this method is often limited by parents' inability to tolerate the baby's apparent hunger and the baby's crying. Unfortunately, rushing back to regular diet can cause a relapse of the vomiting. Following this described regimen, and after at least 24 hours, I would use a mixture of ½ tea and ½ milk (or formula) in the amount and interval which was successfully retained when the tea was last given. From this point on, there should be a gradual return to regular diet which may take a total of 3 to 5 days.

This is a completely physiological approach. It is not a drug, it is not a foreign substance, and it has no side or toxic effects. It can be used in conjunction with any medication prescribed by your doctor. But keep in touch with your doctor.

Diarrhea

In approaching diarrhea, we can use a similar philosophy. First of all, we must consider all serious possibilities, although in most cases there are no serious diseases connected with it. If there is any question— ask your doctor. If it is a simple bowel upset, we again recommend the use of weak, sweet tea. Since the child is not vomiting, we infer that the stomach will tolerate regular doses of liquids so we give as much weak sweet tea as the child will take and tolerate. The objective is the same as that in vomiting: to replace fluids, to replace sugar and to provide a coating of tannic acid for the bowel. The amount of tea given is not limited unless vomiting occurs; however, the diet should completely limited to just this intake and a pattern similar to that in vomiting carried out over the next 4 to 5 day recovery period.

One infection deserves special mention because a vaccine for it has become available. It is called Rotavirus, and has its most serious effect on children three months to two years of age. Usually, there is accompanying fever, nausea or vomiting and it is blamed for many outbreaks of diarrhea especially in nurseries and day-care centers. No antibiotic is effective against Rotavirus so hygienic measures are needed to prevent infection, such as hand-washing and separation from others who may have the illness. Most important is that infants should be immunized as soon as your doctor recommends it, probably early in infancy.

While in every case the ultimate judge and authority for the treatment for the child should be your physician, for the most part, simple vomiting and simple diarrhea do not require any sort of medications, and many of the medications used for these two complaints can have potential dangerous side-effects.

A reminder to parents: If you are administering home treatment and there is a recurrence during or shortly after treatment, or the symptoms persist or increase, call your doctor! Do not persist with home treatment unless there is complete success in a day or two.

Bellyache

We have chosen to use the common term "bellyache" because it is better understood and technically covers more area of the child's body, since it includes the abdominal area as well as the stomach area.

Bellyache is one of the commonest of childhood complaints, and one of the most perplexing. Even for physicians, it presents an extremely difficult diagnosis to make, often exasperating. Everything from emotional upset to stress to mild dysfunction to severe and life-threatening complexes can be the cause.

We have included it, even though there is no common treatment, because there is an inherent warning: Any bellyache, whatever the location, severity, accompanying symptoms, duration, persistence or any other parameter, should be seen by your physician, unless he or she has already advised you about it. Do not delay. Do not self-treat. Certainly, severe or persistent symptoms, or even mild recurrent discomfort should indicate an immediate consultation with your child's physician. This is not the place for "natural products" or over-the-counter medications or home-diagnosis.

SPECIAL MEDICATIONS SITUATIONS

In medicine, there are hundreds of situations in which there are special dangers or urgencies that command the attention of the physician and the respect of the patients. They involve life-threatening situations for the most part. Mostly, they are not for this book.

However, three of them are relatively frequent occurrences and often "at home" situations. We have included them, not to substitute parental care for physician care, but to add some background information relative to the medications used and to increase your understanding, for these illnesses may be chronic.

Diabetes Mellitus

Diabetes is actually more of a disease of adults but sufficient numbers of children do have it to make it important, and it is so much more difficult to treat in children. In fact, children most often have "brittle" diabetes, meaning they are susceptible to minor changes and react more severely than with non-brittle diabetes.

Diabetes is universally known as a disorder of sugar metabolism in which the body cannot deal normally with sugar because of a deficiency of insulin secreted by the pancreas. It is affected by a number of things including exercise, sugar intake, illness and infections. All of these make even more important the basic tenets of diabetes: Insufficient insulin allows the blood sugar to rise and it can reach deadly levels; on the other hand, too much insulin (or too little sugar) creates a dangerous and almost immediate life-threatening situation (called insulin shock). Because of the subtle balances, the calibration of treatment cannot be left to parents or lay people unless they have been carefully trained by the physician or the physician's staff and have been given clearance to make certain judgments. Minute variations in the administration of insulin or insulin-substitutes can be disastrous.

Diabetes treatment in children must be determined by and dictated by the physician, perhaps with the assistance of a diabetes counselor/educator, and the full cooperation of parents. Then, the meticulous care by the parents becomes important to the child.

Asthma

Asthma is a recurrent acute respiratory distress caused by a closing down of the mechanism which allows air to exit from the lungs. Therefore, the child has difficulty breathing and is in a state of panic. Pinning down the causative factors is quite difficult although many of these children are set off by some allergic factor.

It does not usually correct itself and must have medical treatment—mostly emergency care. Without, it, the results may be dire: blood oxygen levels may drop, important chemistries in the body may be altered, and respiratory problems may worsen. On the other hand, too much therapy or the wrong therapy may easily throw the child into other problems. As with diabetes, the sensitive balance between disease and treatment is so delicate that it must be monitored by the physician at all times. There is no room in this disease—either the acute attack or any symptom-free intervals—for parents to manage the child, unless instructed by the doctor.

Medications used may vary including epinephrine, theophylline, other prescribed medications, intravenous fluids, controlled oxygen and other modes. Sometimes, it is necessary to resort to the use of steroids, but never without supervision and constant concern for side effects. Because of the complexity in determining the correct therapy, all decisions must be left to the physician.

Emergencies and shock

There are some situations in childhood that are medical emergencies or in which shock is potentially life-threatening. Shock may be considered a sudden, life-threatening collapse of all body systems and can occur with severe trauma or unresponsive medical conditions. These all require immediate care from your child's doctor or the emergency room.

Some children are highly allergic to certain specific things: bee stings, other insect bites and certain foods. If they are, the children may react with some degree of shock. These extreme reactors need to be carefully monitored—and treated between attacks—and parents have to be trained and prepared for the emergency therapy. In some instances, physicians allow parents to keep an emergency kit of epinephrine (Adrenalin) on hand with instructions on how to use it. Other than this specific order of the physician, all care and prescribing must be done by a physician.

The rule for all three of these potentially-dangerous illnesses is simple. See your doctor immediately-—or another doctor if yours is not available. Do not home treat. Do not manipulate medication. Seek professional help in all instances.

Chapter Seven

HOW TO GIVE MEDICINE TO CHILDREN: EYES, EARS AND NOSE

EYE MEDICATIONS

There are essentially two kinds of eye medication: liquid eye drops and eye ointments. How you instill medication in your child's eye depends on the type of medication and on the age of your child.

Eye Drops

In all cases, your objective is to have the medication reach all parts of the surface of the eyeball and the under-surface of the eyelids. In order to do this, you should place the drops on the eyeball at the outer corner of the eye—there is good reason for this. In the normal structure and function of the eye, tears are released from the tear ducts, which are located near the outer corner of each eye. The normal flow of the tears is from that outer corner to the inner corner where the tears are drained off through a connection with the nose known as the naso-lacrimal duct. Therefore, if drops are placed in the *inner* corner of the eye, the medication will be immediately and directly washed away into that duct, instead of flowing across the entire eye from outer corner to inner corner and the eye will not he bathed with the medicine. The therapeutic effect will be diminished. So, to get the therapeutic effect, the drops should follow the course of tears, from the outer corner, across the eyeball, to the inner corner.

Several general measures are important in the use of eye drops. They are support measures. When there is any discomfort in the eye, moist applications may be applied to the lid of the closed eye several times a day to give your child added comfort, in addition to any eye medication. The external compress applications may be warm (mild) or cool, depending on the tolerance of the child, Simply soak a clean washcloth, wring out the excess water and apply it externally to your child's eye or eyes. No pressure is needed and the eye should be kept closed. Do this for 3 to 5 minutes at a time, anywhere from every hour to every 3 hours, depending on how uncomfortable your child is. If the discomfort continues in spite of this treatment, call your physician.

Before each installation of the drops, the outer surface of the eyelid should be wiped clean with water on absorbent cotton in order to remove any excess pus or crusting on the outside of the lid. The moist cotton should be wiped once very gently across the closed eyelid or down the closed eyelid to wipe the excess material away. Use a clean cotton ball every time you wipe the eye.

Always keep the dropper clean. If the dropper is part of a dropper bottle, replacing it in the bottle without touching it to the eye or any other surface will help it remain sterile. If the dropper you are using is separate from the bottle, be sure to wash it each time in running water, especially immediately before using the drops, and be careful that it does not touch any other surface.

If the drops need to be stored in a refrigerator, let them come up to room temperature before you use them.

Positioning the Child

For Older Children

Usually, the child should be lying down for the administration of the drops. If the child is older and very cooperative, the drops may be placed in the eye while the child tilts his or her head backward. He or she can be in a sitting or a standing position.

For Infants and Younger Children

Remember that small children will always object to lying still and will vigorously fight being restrained. In addition, they may be uncomfortable or frightened. This often makes it difficult to instill drops, but calm and loving persistence of the parents will help ease the child and you will succeed in getting the drops in the eye.

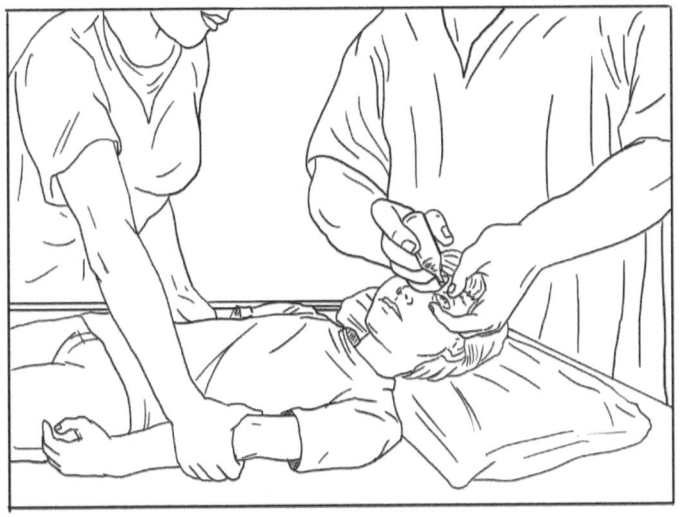

Figure 3

Drops should always be instilled in the eye with the small child lying on his or her back. In order to achieve the greatest success, a two-person approach is probably best (Figure 3). One adult immobilizes the child by controlling the child's body: leaning over the child as he or she lies on a flat surface, pinning the arms to the side or holding the arms and seeing that the legs do not kick. The other adult then separates the eyelids using his or her thumb and forefinger of the same hand and instills the drops in the outer corner of the eye with the other hand. This should be done as swiftly as possible, but without trauma and without touching the eye dropper to the eye at any time— or creating an emotional scene that upsets the child more.

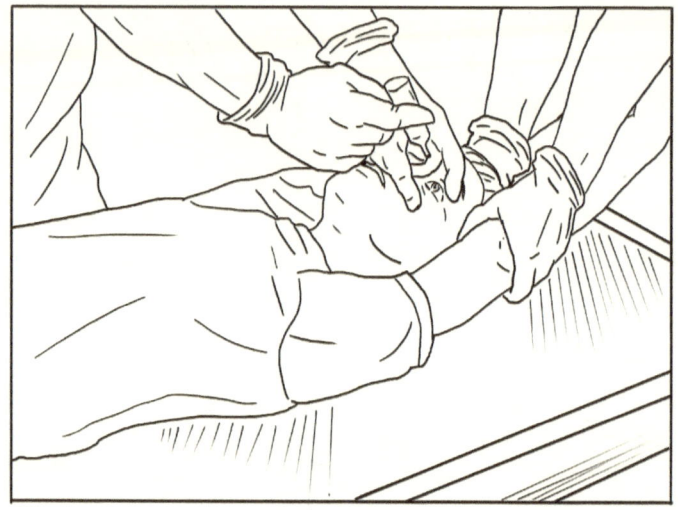

Figure 4

Here's another two-person restraint technique (Figure 4): Lay the child on a table or bed. With the child's arms held out straight over his or her head, one adult presses the child's elbows against the child's head and immobilizes the child's arms and head in that one maneuver. Evading any kicking the child maybe doing, the second adult instills the drops.

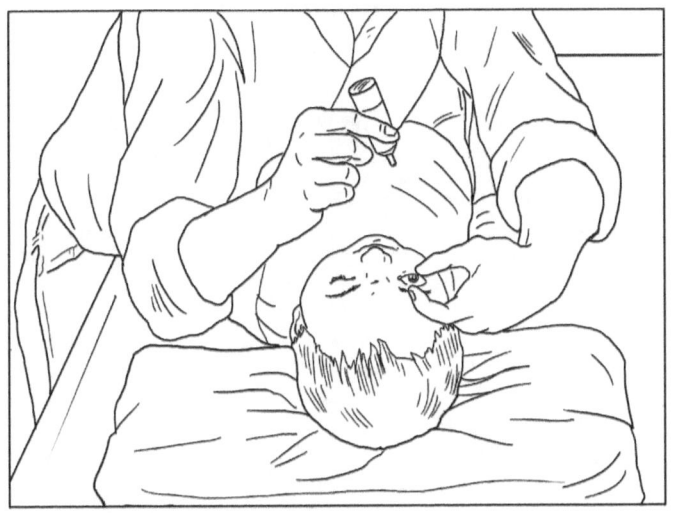

Figure 5

If you are doing this alone, it becomes more tricky (Figure 5). It is possible, with practice, to lay the child down in front of you on a table or bed, lean over him and pin his arms to his sides with your elbows, leaving your hands free for instilling the drops. If you are right-handed, use your left hand to keep the head from rolling from side to side, and the thumb and forefinger of that left hand to hold the lids apart. The right hand should hold the dropper if you are right-handed. Use the side of the right palm to hold the baby's head steady and place the drops in the outer corner of the eye.

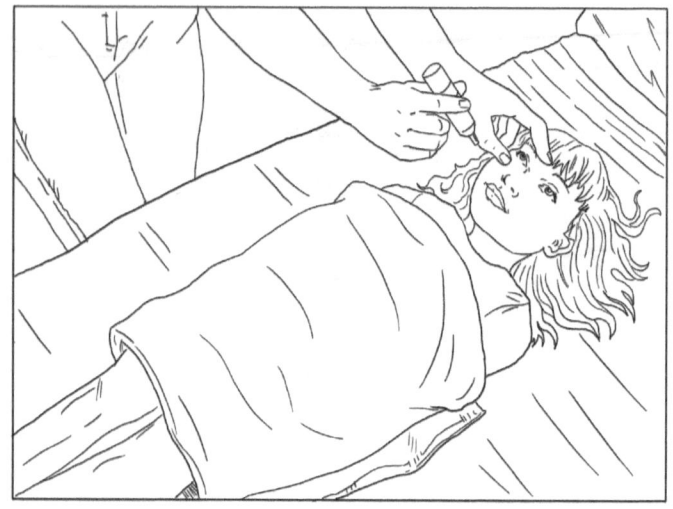

Figure 6

Another technique is available for the struggling, kicking, squirming, crying child but it basically is for the infant or toddler (Figure 6). It can be used either with one adult or two. Place your child on his or her back on a bath towel with the length of the towel at right angles to the body. Reasonably tightly, cross one end of the towel across the baby's chest to his other side. Now cross the opposite corner of the towel over the child and wrap excess toweling under the child. This should immobilize the child. DO NOT COVER THE CHILD'S FACE OR TIGHTEN THE TOWEL ACROSS THE NECK AND DO NOT LET THE TOWEL INTERFERE WITH BREATHING! With this procedure, instilling of eye drops (or nose drops or ear drops), should be much easier. Try to help the child avoid too much blinking as this hastens loss of medication from the eye and therefore decreases effectiveness of the drops.

Eye Ointments

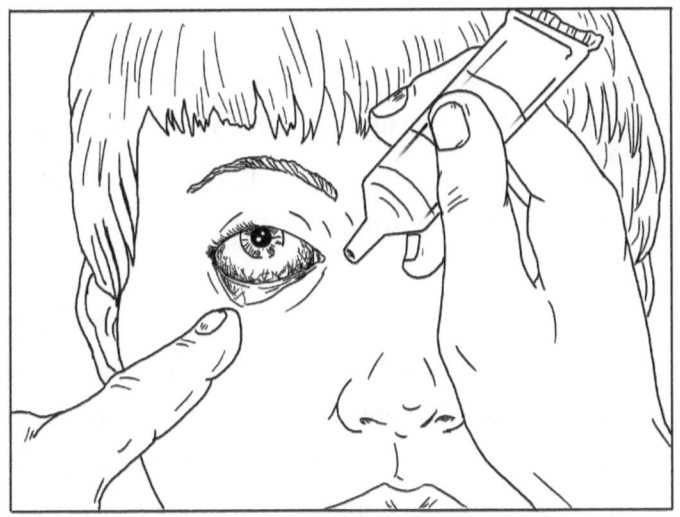

Figure 7

In all children, the idea is to pull down the lower lid until it is turned outward far enough for you to see the red or pink conjunctiva (inner lining of the lid) (Figure 7). Squeeze from the ointment tube to the inner surface of the eyelid approximately ¼ to 1/2 inch of the medication. Be careful not to touch the tube to the child's eye or hold it so close that a sudden movement will make it touch the eye or poke it. Immediately close the eyelid with your fingers and very gently rub them over the external eyelid in a circular motion once or twice.

The importance of immobilizing the child in order to prevent any damage and to be certain of applying the medicine properly is the same for both types of medications. Always remember that you are dealing with a very delicate, easily-injured structure. Take time. Take care. Preventing injury or damage is every bit as important as applying the medicine.

Sometimes drops or ointments can be placed in the eye while the child is asleep, especially if he or she is a deep sleeper. Always remember to be certain the child is restrained anyway, because sudden awakening or unexpected movement could cause damage.

NASAL MEDICATION

Nose Drops

The best position for administering nose drops is for the child to be lying on his or her back with the head bent slightly backwards. Sometimes this can be better achieved by putting the child's shoulders on a pillow and letting the head tilt back toward the surface. You can control the body of a struggling infant or child the same as you do for eye drops.

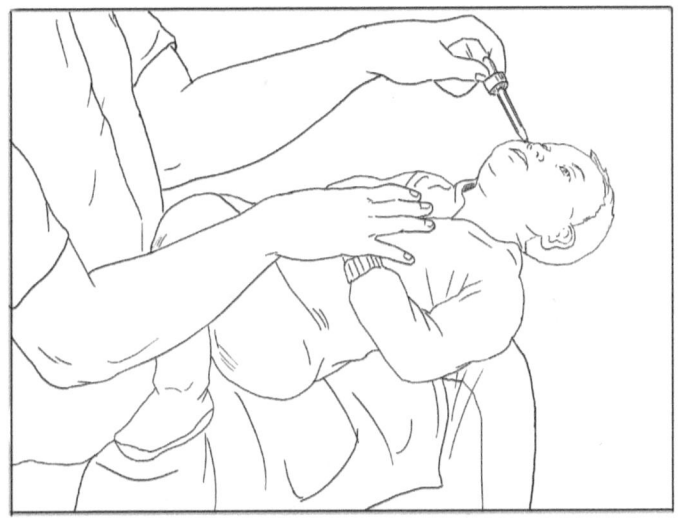

Figure 8

With a smaller infant who is struggling and resisting, you might try this positioning (Figure 8): With the parent sitting, place the baby on its back on the parent's lap, with the head away from the parent's body. Allow the baby's head to drop slightly toward the floor between or over the parent's knees. Using one hand to control the baby's arms, use the other hand to instill the drops.

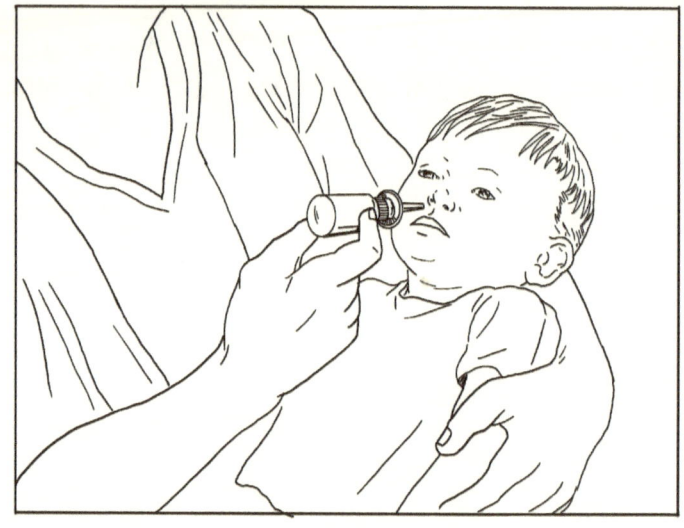

Figure 9

For small infants, you should place the baby with its head in the crook of your arm with his closest arm behind your back (Figure 9). Your one arm should firmly hold his free arm with his body against you, while your opposite hand places the drops in the nose.

Whenever possible, the child's nose should be cleared before putting in drops. Never put any rigid objects in the nose to clean it, such as Q-tips or applicators—at any time. If the nose is very stuffy so that it seems occluded, clearing it as we describe below may be difficult but should be tried. Older children may assist by blowing their noses,—clearing out mucus or exudate. For the younger child, parents should use a bulb syringe to suction out the mucus *gently.* When the mucus is very thick, instill the salt-baking soda mixture (described under Common Treatments for Common Problems in Chapter *5)* or a plain salt water solution, a few drops in each nostril. Then you may suck out the contents of the nose with the bulb syringe, inserting the tip of the bulb syringe just inside the nares (outer opening of the nose). Do not push the tip any further than this!

In instilling the nose drops, the prescribed amount should be put in each nostril without the dropper itself touching the child's nose, if possible. This avoids picking up any infectious material on the dropper. The child should remain lying flat for about *3-5* minutes after installation of the drops, if possible. If the dropper accidentally does touch the child's nose (or anything else), wash the dropper carefully (running water is fine) before returning it to the bottle.

When treating a very stuffy nose, it sometimes helps to instill one drop of the prescribed medication in each nostril initially, then wait about a minute, so that the inner tissues nearest the opening of the nose have been relieved of some of the congestion. Then put the remaining drop or two or three (depending on the prescription) into each nostril. This will allow medication to penetrate to the upper part of the lining of the nose, for more effective relief, without being obstructed. Remember to have older children blow their noses before using the drops, or in the younger child, use a bulb syringe as described to clear out any mucus.

For the most part, the majority of physicians recommend against using sprays in children as this is liable to force infected material up into the nose or even into the sinuses. Unless ordered by a physician, sprays should not be used in children. It may appear to parents to be easier but it is less effective and carries some danger.

Additional hints: If the drops are over-the-counter medication, do not use them for more than five days, or stop if the child's condition worsens before then. Use them only according to the labeled directions. If it is a prescription, follow your physician's instructions.

EAR MEDICATIONS

Ear Drops

Ear drops should always be administered with the child in a horizontal position with the ear to be treated facing upward. If the child is an infant or toddler and is resisting, a holding pattern can be used (as in eye and ear administration). If the drops have been refrigerated, they should be allowed to come up to room temperature.

Putting your child on his or her back with the head turned to the side should place the ear canal in an approximately vertical position. The ear drops should be dropped into the ear canal opening so that they may drop down by gravity into the canal itself. (do not squirt!). If needed, a small cotton ball may be applied afterward to the external opening of the ear to avoid the medicine spilling out when the child gets up.

Ear drops must be able to reach the ear drum by gravity in order for the medication to be effective. How easily they reach the drum is affected by the direction the ear canal takes from the outer ear to the drum. Actually, it goes in one anatomical direction in children under about 3 years of age and goes in a different direction after that as the child grows. Thus, instructions for instilling drops will be slightly different in the two age-groups:

Children Under Three Years of Age

The bottom of the earlobe should be gently pulled downward (towards the child's shoulder) and backward (toward the back of the child's head) while instilling the drops. This will allow the drops to flow freely into the canal.

Children Over Three Years of Age

Holding the ear at the top of the ear lobe, it should be pulled gently upward (toward the top of the child's head) and backward (toward the back of the child's head). Keeping the ear in this position, drop the medication into the opening without letting the dropper touch the ear.

Remember—ear pulled *downward and backward* in small children but *upward and backward* for those over 3 years of age.

The earlobe should then be very gently moved back and forth once or twice, so that the fluid will enter the ear properly. Keep the child in the same position for a few minutes so that the drops can get to the affected area.

Keep the outside of the canal as dry as possible between instillation of drops. NEVER insert any rigid objects into the canal, such as Q-tips, swabs, applicators or any other cleaning device. Use soft absorbent cotton, only as far as it fits comfortably.

Ear ointments and creams

When the *wall* of the canal is being treated (as with skin infection in the ear canal or eczema in the canal, for example), the physician might order an ear wick to hold the medication against the canal wall. To make a wick for the ear, take a small wisp or segment or strand of dry absorbent cotton, roll it into a small cylinder with your fingers. It should be about one inch long and 1/16" in thickness. Using any of the holding techniques, gently insert the dry wick into the ear canal, holding the ear according to age, as described above, always leaving enough cotton outside the ear to be able to remove it easily. Inserting this wick will be somewhat difficult because it is so flexible! Do not use any rigid objects to put it in the ear. Gently persist, perhaps moving the canal to get a straighter entry. When the wick is in place, drop the medication on the outside (exposed) area of cotton to soak it—usually 3 drops will be sufficient.

If your doctor orders ointment, place a thin layer of the ointment on the wick before inserting it, then gently slide the wick into the ear canal. The wick, now soaked with medication, will press the medicine against the canal wall for constant application. Leave it in place as prescribed by your physician.

Chapter Eight

HOW TO ADMINISTER MEDICINES BY MOUTH TO CHILDREN

Giving oral medication to your children can be complicated by their age, their maturity and their cooperativeness. Thus, you must know different methods of administration for different stages of life and development. How you give oral medicine also depends on the form and type of the prescription ordered by the doctor.

When you are ready to administer medication, first put everything you will need together in one place near the child—medication, spoon, dropper, bib, towel, follow-up drink and anything else of importance. This prevents your needing to leave in the middle of the procedure to get a missing item.

Parents and doctors have several concerns in dealing with oral medication:

Accurate dosage. In every type of medication, the dosage delivered to the child must be accurate. Problems can occur if dosage is incorrect.

Irritation of the mucous membrane lining of the stomach. Certain medications, by their nature, are irritants to the stomach and can cause not only discomfort but might also cause actual ulceration. Choosing the proper form of the oral medication is important.

Child's ability to swallow. If the ability of your child to swallow is interfered with in any way, either by disease or other factors, or because of age, your child will probably not be able to swallow solid medication. Therefore, liquid medication will probably be preferred.

Speed of effect. You must always remember that, for the most part, medication put into the stomach must ultimately be absorbed into the bloodstream (either in the stomach or in the intestine), and then distributed by way of the bloodstream to the rest of the body. That's why this route of administration is slower than injection (whether under the skin or into a muscle)—and much slower than direct injection into blood stream. The effects of injected medication are usually seen shortly after administration; even some topical medication may have a faster time of action than oral medication. Depending on the medication, the condition of the child and the forms in which the medication is manufactured, your doctor will choose which speed of action is needed. Not all medications can be used by all routes.

Taste and acceptance. If a medicine is bitter, or has an odd feel in the child's mouth, or for some reason is not acceptable to a child, the medication will not be taken. (For example, a medicine may be cherry-flavored and some children may not like cherry). Consequently, there will be no therapeutic effect. Manufacturers of pharmaceuticals try to make medication in the most acceptable form or forms but sometimes their efforts have to be supplemented by your ingenuity as a parent.

Today, many pharmacies will compound your child's medication with the flavor of that child's choice, making it more acceptable.

Acceptance by the child. Children often resist taking oral medication—some mildly and some violently. Following the suggestions later in this chapter and the next one may help greatly to minimize these reactions. However, if the resistance or reaction is overwhelming and exaggerated, consult your child's physician about this behavior. There may be more than one cause for it.

UNDERSTANDING ORAL MEDICATION

Oral medications can be in several forms, often reflecting the type of medication and its purpose. Oral medication comes is either solid or liquid form.

Liquid Medication

As indicated before, liquid medication is much easier for small children to take than solid form. At very young ages, it is the only form of oral medication which can be used. Probably for those under the age of 5 years, liquid medication—if available—is preferable to solid medication. Read the label every time you give a dose, and do not confuse tablespoon with teaspoon; most doses are in teaspoon amounts.

There are different types of liquid medication for small children. These types need to be understood:

Elixirs. Certain medications dissolve more completely in a liquid that contains some alcohol. These are called elixirs. Over-the-counter elixirs should never be given to children, because of the alcohol content. Doctors, of course, will be wary of prescribing medication that comes only in elixir form but there are instances in which this is needed, and the doctor should decide.

Syrups. Syrups are solutions with a high sugar content and many liquid medicines come in syrup form. The sugar helps to disguise an unpleasant taste. Although for most children the amount of sugar in a syrup should not have any bad effect, consideration has to be given to children who are diabetic, or those who have sugar sensitivity or those to whom you do not wish to administer extra sugar intake, for whatever reason.

Suspensions. There are solid medications which do not dissolve in common liquids (such as water, syrup or elixir) but will "float" in those or in some other liquid. However, because the medication is not dissolved, only suspended ("floating") in the fluid, the medical substance tends to settle out in the mixture, so that after standing for a little while, the medicine at the bottom of the bottle will be much more concentrated and yield a heavier dose than at the top of the bottle. Hence, the instruction, "Shake well before using." This is extremely important and suspensions should be vigorously shaken *immediately* before administering the medication to the child. Even this does not guarantee accurate and consistent doses, but is the best that can be done for certain medications.

The danger in this situation is that if a child gets a dilute dose (as it would be early in the use of unshaken medication), he or she will have less than adequate therapeutic effect. If the medication continues to be concentrated at the bottom of the bottle (because of failure to shake the bottle), the "bottom" doses from that bottle will be concentrated, giving the child too heavy a dose and perhaps bringing on a toxic effect. Phenytoin (Dilantin) Suspension, a very effective drug for epilepsy and seizures, is an example of what has been described, and there have been reports in the literature of severely toxic effects of Dilantin in children for whom the suspension was needed but where parents or others failed to shake the bottle sufficiently.

Liquid medication is dispensed by spoon or dropper and one of the most challenging things to do in the administration of liquid medication is to measure the dosage accurately and consistently. It takes effort on the part of the parent, even though the dosage as prescribed and sold is generally uniform.

Dropper. Medication is administered by dropper (usually with a dropper bottle) when the dose is smaller than a teaspoonful, as it may be for an infant, or for when the dosage must be measured in drops or other minute amounts because of the concentration or critical nature of the medication. Never switch a dropper from one medication to another without cleaning it thoroughly first. Better, never switch droppers.

Spoon. This is the route used for most oral medications. But there are problems. The ordinary household teaspoon is not an accurate delivery vehicle for medication as household teaspoons vary greatly in their content. There is no guarantee your teaspoon meets the standard for accurate measure of a teaspoon. Some landmark work has been done showing that the actual contents of household teaspoons fail to be consistent and may hold anywhere from 2.5 cubic centimeters to almost 10 cubic centimeters, depending also in part on how much the spoon is filled and what the fluid is.

Officially, when the directions specify a teaspoon, that means 5 cubic centimeters (cc) of fluid. That is what the physician means and it is so dispensed by the pharmacist. So when the doctor says, "Give one teaspoonful," it means the delivery of 5 cubic centimeters (cc) of the medication, so as to ensure the proper dose. There can also be major differences in content when different persons fill the same teaspoon. Differences have even been found with the same person using the same teaspoon because of variations in the amount of filling of the spoon.

Fortunately, there are on the market, but too infrequently used, a number of devices for accurately measuring liquid drugs, including special measuring spoons, medication cups and, particularly, droppers. One of the best is the oral syringe (no needle), which probably gives the most accurate measurement because the amounts are clearly marked. Dosage amounts are read from those markings on the syringe. The medication can be dropped into the baby's mouth or the child's mouth directly from the oral syringe with an exact dose. Be sure to place the tip of the syringe inside the cheek (remember the syringe has no needle attached) and at the side of the tongue (not in the middle or directed toward the throat). Then, gently push the plunger so that the medication goes into the mouth. If the amount is large, squirt just a small amount in, wait for the child to swallow and then squirt a little more in. We recommend that all parents purchase an accurate measuring device before it becomes necessary to administer medication; it will save aggravation later. Consult your pharmacist about his suggestion for your child and have him demonstrate its use.

In using these measuring devices, be sure to clean them thoroughly after each use, When it is necessary for someone else to administer the medicine (teacher, school nurse, neighbor), be certain to pass the measuring device on to them, and, if necessary, explain the use of it.

Bad-tasting medication is one of the major problems in oral medication. Manufacturers always try to disguise the taste within the bounds of other restrictions but are not always as successful as they—and we—would like. So we occasionally find ourselves trying to administer to our children medicines that are distasteful to them.

Parents can help by trying several things. First, try the medication as manufactured. Some children may not find it objectionable; what is 'good" to one may be 'ugh" to another. If the child finds it distasteful, however, even if others find it satisfactory, try to disguise it.

It is permissible to offer something sweet to a child to get him or her to take the medication. One method is to give the child, if he or she is old enough, a "sweet", such as chocolate bud, gum drop or jelly bean, immediately after the dose of medicine. This may take away the bitter taste or minimize it, or it may become an incentive to overlook the taste. The child may even look forward to this treat when the next dose of the medication arrives or at least be more receptive.

Another method is to disguise directly the taste of the medication. This usually works when the treat does not, or when the child is too young for a solid treat. For example, measure the usual dose of one teaspoonful (measured exactly) and put it into a tablespoon, then add a drop or two of chocolate syrup or strawberry juice or cranberry juice or apple juice. If this makes it more palatable for the child, continue; if not, add a little more of the special sweetener the next time and do this until the child accepts the medication. Other substances used to disguise taste include honey, sugar water or maple syrup. Do not use large quantities of the sweet flavoring and do not put the medication into a glass with large amounts of a sweetened substance. If the child does not take it all, he or she therefore will not get the full dose of medication. Check with your pharmacist to be sure the flavoring will not interfere with the absorption or effectiveness of the medication.

Two precautions for both these methods: First, do not do this with diabetic children because the sugar will add a glucose load which may affect the child. Second, be extremely careful that, if the "bad" taste does come through, it does not destroy the child's interest in and taste for the chocolate syrup or strawberry or whatever you are using. Once more, today's pharmacies will often flavor the medication to your child's taste.

Two additional precautions. Never tell a child that the medicine tastes good and never tell a child that it is candy. And do not punish the child's fussing; instead, sympathize with the child.

Solid Medication

For adults, of course, the administration of solid medication, such as tablets and capsules, is very simple. So it is for older children and adolescents. They merely swallow the tablet whole and the process is over.

The two options available in using solid medication for smaller children are chewing the entire table (when it can be chewed) or swallowing the table whole. When a lesser dose is needed and there is no liquid form, cutting the table in half may be necessary—and you will be told so by your physician or pharmacist. In other instances, crushing the dose into some other solid substance, for example, applesauce, or dissolving it in water or juice are available avenues. The method used depends upon the type of medication, the dosage required, and the maturity or acceptance of the child. But never divide a tablet in less than half because the accuracy of the dose will be affected.

Solid medication may be administered in several different ways:

Swallowing the entire tablet. This is only for children old enough to swallow a tablet intact and where the full tablet is the correct dosage.

Chewing the tablet. Tablets should not be chewed unless there is a direction on the prescription or on the over-the-counter medication indicating that it is satisfactory to do so. If you are uncertain, check with your pharmacist first. Otherwise, do not allow your child to chew a tablet or capsule.

In order to decrease the number and frequency of doses of certain medicines, manufacturers have devised long-acting (L.A.) or sustained-release (SR) tablets. These tablets are identified (either on the tablet or on the prescription bottle) as long-acting (L.A.) or sustained release (SR) or are accompanied by a warning on the label. Sometimes they are given other designations. Medication usually requiring an every four-hour dose can be sometimes built into a special tablet that gives an even release of the medication into the body over an eight-hour or twelve-hour or 24-hour period. When the manufacturer uses a special construction of the tablet, the release of some medicine from the tablet into the child's system is slowed down and distributed evenly over the longer period of time. Disturbing the structure of a long-acting tablet destroys its slow-release capabilities, and may put the 8-hour or 12-hour or 24-hour dose into the child's system all at once. Therefore, the slow-acting tablet must *never* be cut or chewed or crushed. Overdose of the medicine can occur, with great potential dangers. Again, your pharmacist can advise you.

Crushing the tablet. When a child cannot swallow a tablet or chew it whole, the tablet (if it is not L.A. or SR) may be crushed very carefully and completely. If your pharmacist says the tablet may be crushed, place it in a dry tablespoon. Put a teaspoon on top of the tablespoon, hold the bowls of the two spoons, press and grind them together and then mix it into any substance acceptable to the child. Sometimes apple sauce or ice cream will work. This mixture is then fed to the child as would-be regular food. The favorite mediums for crushed tablets are applesauce (because of its universal acceptance in children and babies), chocolate pudding (because of its wide acceptance and sweet taste), jelly, jam, ice cream, chocolate syrup or similar substances. It is wise to continue to search for a substance the child will accept. Sometimes it helps to let the child choose which he or she prefers. Generally, the tablet should not be placed in liquids, such as milk, water or soda, because it may not dissolve or it may impart a bad taste and perhaps may spoil the child's taste for that liquid later.

Several rules apply when you give medication in a disguising substance:

- There should be enough of the disguising substance to hide the taste of the medication.

- There should not be a large amount of the substance either, because if the child fails to take the total volume, he or she will get a lesser dose and lose the therapeutic effect.

- Care should be taken that the medication does not change the child's enjoyment of the disguising substance. It is probably better to use an unfamiliar liquid (prune juice, for example) rather than a familiar and enjoyable one (milk, for example).

- The medication in the disguising substance should be given before meals or when the child would appear to be hungry (avoiding after meals when the child is full and may not take the medication with the substance).

115

Be sure that this does not interfere with your doctor's prescribed instructions.

• Never use this as a means of dividing a tablet into several doses.

• Be careful not to make the disguising substance so attractive that the child will confuse it with a confection—especially if the mixture stands around the house freely.

Dissolving the tablet. You should do this only on instruction of the doctor or the pharmacist as all tablets do not dissolve. One of those professionals should tell you what kind of liquid in which to dissolve the medication. Most frequently used are water, sweet tea, and fruit juice. The same precautions apply as in crushing the tablet and you should be very careful to observe those guidelines.

Cutting the tablet in half. There are instances in which the dosage ordered for the child is not manufactured by the pharmaceutical company and it is necessary to take a larger tablet and divide it in half. Unless the tablet is scored (has an indentation down the center of the tablet for ease of breaking), you should not attempt to cut tablets in half. You most likely will not get equality of doses, and also may wind up wasting a good bit of the medication, which means the child will not get a sufficient dose. Your pharmacist may be able to help by dividing the tablets for you. If you are going to need to divide tablets more than a couple of times, ask the pharmacist about an inexpensive tablet cutter. There are several efficient ones on the market and the pharmacist can show you how to use it.

The precautions for long-acting tablets, described under *Chewing the tablet* applies equally to crushing, dissolving and cutting a long-acting tablet in half. These should not be done.

Swallowing the entire tablet, chewing it or crushing it should be used only when the dosage ordered is the entire tablet. Cutting the tablet in half is done only when the prescribed dose is exactly half of the tablet dispensed. You should never crush tablets in an attempt to give the child half or a third of the dose; it will not work and the child will get the wrong dose.

Not everything solid is a tablet There are capsules, gelatin capsules (soft and usually colored), coated and other forms. These can not be crushed or dissolved. Refer any problems or questions to your pharmacist.

Once a child learns to swallow a pill whole, the rest is easy but there is a transition or learning period for each child—for some a short time and for some a long time. This, as we pointed out, should be reserved for children who are physically and psychologically prepared to do this, preferable over the age of 5 years. The child should first take a small sip of fluid (such as fruit juice, water or tea), hold it in his or her mouth, then immediately put the pill/tablet/capsule between his/her closed lips and then swallow the rest of the fluid at once. This will then wash the medication down into the esophagus. If the child coughs or chokes, stop the procedure at once.

Medication should always be given as your doctor or pharmacist instructs. Try not to miss any doses, do not give any extra doses and always finish the complete prescription, unless your physician instructs you otherwise.

Part Three

MANAGING THE CHILD

Chapter Nine

SPECIAL PRECAUTIONS

Always check with your doctor or pharmacist before giving over-the-counter medications, especially if your child is already taking some other medication.

Medications, whether liquid or solid, should never be made attractive to the child. The parents' dilemma is to have the child accept the medication yet not think of it as a treat. Parents have been known to tell the child that the medication is candy or that it was a special treat, or make the administration of it so sweet and flavorful that that the child might seek it when it was not needed. This is a difficult dilemma for a parent.

Your first caution is *always* to keep medications out of the reach of children, but it is best if you keep it in locked cabinets. Always use child-resistant caps. Then, explain to the child that the medication is being given to make him feel better and to get rid of his illness. It should be further explained that medication is *not* to be taken at any other time because it can have the reverse effect: it can make you sick.

The child should clearly understand (because some of them do make this mistake) that the medication is *not* being given as any form of punishment or because the child was bad. The child should never feel that his illness, that is, his cough or tummy ache, was a punishment for something that he or she did wrong. A not-unusual scenario is the child who develops a cold and is told by a parent, "See, I told you not to go out in the rain and now you have this cold and I had to take you to the doctor and you have to take this medicine." Children take parents' words at their exact meaning and a child in this situation is liable to conjure up visions of his symptoms being the punishment for disobeying mother and the medication as a further punishment. This interferes with the realistic acceptance of the medication for what it is. It also undermines the child's confidence in the parent and interferes with the parent-child relationship. After any episode of administering medication, whether drops or ointments or oral drugs, if your child is crying or upset or angry, you should soothe the child, proffer love and show complete acceptance. Hugs, applauding and praising are always in order. A child should never be made to feel guilty about being upset by those procedures. "I understand and I love you" carries great weight and helps a great deal in resolving some of these problems.

Sometimes the parents' attitude will interfere with the child's acceptance of medication, both oral and instillations into eyes, ears or nose. If you approach the child apologizing or profusely explaining or looking as though you expect a battle with the medication, the likelihood is that you will have a battle. At times there are parental conversations which prepare the child to fight. If she hears, "Well it's time for her medicine again. I guess we'll have more screaming and fighting", there will be screaming and fighting.

Be quiet. Be patient. Act confident. No matter how many times you have had resistance, approach the child with an attitude that says, "We are going to be successful this time." Talk calmly to the child about something altogether different when approaching with the medicine. Do not fall into the trap of asking the child whether he or she wants to take the medication. Be firm, but sometimes giving some choice will help, such as "Do you want to take your medicine in the kitchen or the bedroom?" (or "before or after Sesame Street" or "before or after nap time" or "before or after" some other small event in the home.)

Always keep your cool. Do not lose your temper over the medication. Do not get involved in lengthy discussions or debates about the medicine. No screaming or hollering or threatening. You must remain calm no matter how difficult it is—that's what parents are for. Speak in a soft voice, say gentle things, and comfort the child with cuddling or hugging—before, during or after. Often a reward given afterward, like a star on a chart, or a sweet, for example, will make subsequent doses easier.

You should always point out, when necessary—within the child's concepts of understanding—the ultimate goal of taking the medicine: to be able to go back to school, to resume playing sports, to be able to go to the movies or similar incentives. Do not lie about the taste of the medication, and let your children know that you understand their distaste and sympathize with them. If you agree with them say so, but point out the necessity.

You should always let the child know when medicine is being mixed into the food (and when it is not), and praise every success along the way.

If a child rejects or spits out some medication, begin all over again—without fuss. Be careful to see that the child gets the proper amount—and not too much—in case he or she has swallowed some and then you need to administer some more medication to make the proper dose.

One last warning: Very often, parents are confused after they leave the doctor's office and they forget the instructions given them. If this happens to you—even if you've forgotten even just a small detail—be sure to check with your physician or pharmacist before administering the medication.

Chapter Ten

DEVELOPMENTAL CONSIDERATIONS IN ADMINISTERING DRUGS

It is obvious that no mother would give her infant a solid tablet to swallow. Mother knows very well that the development of the infant and his or her age would cause choking and perhaps do serious damage. This is a perfect example of why the administration of medicine to children must be based on the child's sophistication and actual physical development. These developmental landmarks must be guidelines to the administration of medicine and are the reason that physicians will advise mothers how to give the necessary drug so that it can be used by the body in the easiest possible fashion. The child getting nose drops has to be positioned so that the drops can be instilled in an effective manner. Similarly with ear drops and eye drops. In case of oral medication, the form of the medication and the technique of administering must be based on the child's experience and development and on the presence of certain maturity milestones.

In order to obtain cooperation of toddlers and older children, they should always be given some sort of choices in the administration of medication, whenever possible. Do you want to be on the bed or sit on my lap to get your nose drops? Shall we put the ear drops in before or after lunch? Do you want your medicine in apple sauce or in chocolate pudding? Similar choices bring the child into the situation as an active participant. Once the child has helped with the answer, he or she has already accepted being a participant and is taking the first step in cooperation. Infants, or very small children, may take medication more readily if they are cuddled in your arms—they need physical comforting, not just verbal reassurances.

It is impossible to give specific rules for specific ages or certain medications. Managing children, especially during illness, requires some understanding of each particular child's development—what the child is capable of doing or not doing, and how the child tends to react in various situations. Most mothers, consciously or unconsciously, know these parameters. But mothers need to consider those developmental levels in administering medication. Helpful to mothers (and fathers) are a number of good books on child development, especially those that spell out typical developmental levels. These can be used for guidance when a child is ill.

Here are some examples. Infants often will spit out any food, medication or other substance they do not want or like. Knowing this, parents will be extra careful when administering medications. When the child reaches a year of so, you can often successfully use games (you must make them up) to gain the cooperation of the child. This is another helpful hint from a developmental level. Other examples to consider are: the young walker is capable of running away or kicking, and by 2-plus years, children have become very capable of resisting whatever they do not want.

So it pays to take a few moments whenever medication is required to think about the "stage" the child is in, and adjust your approach accordingly.

Epilogue

They are precious and darling. They are our children. And, as such, they deserve the best care. When they are ill, they ought to get a little more attention, and it has been the objective of this book to help parents with the onerous task of understanding medications and the difficult problem of administering medications to children of all ages. If it helped—even a little bit—it was a worthwhile task.

So, GOOD LUCK!

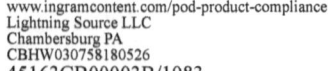